Food Combining

For

Weight Loss

Derek Lee

1

Table of Contents

Introduction...4
Step I...8
Step II...9
Step III...10
Step IV...14
Step V...16
Step VI...17
Step VII..18
 Step VIII...20
Step IX...22
Step X...24

Introduction

Greetings,

Hello! My name is Derek. I am in my mid 30s. Normally, for the past decade, I usually weigh between 140-150 lbs.

In the last year, everything completely changed. Probably because I'm getting older and my metabolism is slowing down. Or perhaps it's because of lack of activity and exercise. Maybe it's just plain laziness. I was shocked when my scale showed 180 lbs. I couldn't believe my eyes.

I've come to realize that the older I am, the harder it is for me to lose weight and have a flat stomach. Instead of just accepting it, I needed to change. I don't want to be obese.

I decided to do change my eating habits. If you're like me, you may have looked into some of the popular diets such as Atkins, Ketogenic, Paleo, etc.

I tried cutting carbohydrates. I tried eating only egg whites. I've tried abstaining from red meats. When it comes to the weight loss programs, I discovered that most of them didn't work. It was a waste of time, effort and lots of money.

After experimenting with many different types of diets, I felt tired, hungry and often bloated. I even tried cleanses like the colon and liver cleanse. Sometimes, I am constipated for a few days. I didn't know the reasons, but it didn't stop me from searching for answers.

In trying to change my diet and eating habits, I've learned that eating the right food was just half the coin. The other half of the coin is about making sure I eat the right foods at the right time. I stumbled on this missing piece of the puzzle. It has to do with food combining.

Proper food combining helps my body to assimilate nutrients for energy and cleanse out waste. If food can't move through the body properly, it becomes overloaded with toxicity, leaving me feeling bad, even though the quality of food I'm eating is good.

With a few simple tweaks to diet, proper food pairing, the results are amazing. I have more energy, better skin, better sleep and natural weight loss within a few days.

What exactly is Food Combining?

Food combining is understanding that different types of foods digest at different rates and with different enzymes. Some foods digest better in an acidic environment, while others digest better in an alkaline environment.

When you eat several foods that digest at different rates, it calls for different enzymes or need different pH levels, your digestion gets out of whack and things begin to rot and ferment in your body.

This "sludge" turns into stored toxins. When your body can't digest food properly, it misses out on being able to absorb the nutrients in food, leaving you with low energy, skin breakouts and poor sleep.

Food combining guidelines take into account the speed at which food digests. Fruit digests the quickest, then greens, then non-starchy vegetables, then starches and finally, digesting the slowest is protein.

Eating foods in the correct order (according to their transit times) ensures a traffic jam-free (and toxin-free) digestive tract.

When you get the combining right, your body gets to use the nutrients in the food. This leaves you with more energy, healthy body and weight loss.

Here are the food combining basics:

Starches + Veggies = OK
Proteins + Veggies = OK
Proteins + Starches = NO
Plant Proteins + Plant Proteins = OK
Animal Proteins + Animal Proteins = NO
Starches + Starches = OK
Fats + Proteins (animal or plant) = NO (or pair moderately)
Fats + Carbohydrates = OK
Fats + Starches = OK
Fruits are best eaten on an empty stomach
Fruit + Raw greens = OK (except melons)

These guidelines may seem overwhelming at first, but it's really quite simple to find meals that work. Let's get on the right track by eliminating a couple of common food combinations and consuming combinations that are good and healthy for the body.

Step I

Imagine yourself on a freeway. You will notice that every car travels differently. Some cars are in the fast lane. Some are observing the recommended speed limit. Some cars are in the slow lane.

Similarly, different types of food or drink take different amounts of time to digest.

Here is the approximate time that it takes to digest:

Water
15 minutes

Juices
30 minutes

Fruit
30 minutes – 1 hour

Vegetables
1hr – 2hrs to digest

Meat and Fish
over 4 hours

Shellfish
over 8 hours

Step II

Combining Food is like a marriage relationship.

Some marriage relationships are compatible. Other relationships may work for a short period of time, but in the long run, it will not last. It will be detrimental to the entire family system.

For example, avocado and tomato goes very well together. But don't combine beans and cheese (any type of dairy).

By trying different types of food combinations, you can see which one works for you.

Although there are generic similarities with all people, however, every person is unique and different. Some people have allergic reactions to certain types of food.

Our stomachs digest differently depending upon our age, health, history and genetic makeup.

Despite these different factors, there are certain commonalities among all people. It will take some experimentation and trial and error on your part. But eventually, you'll figure out which food combinations works the best.

Step III

Fruits are good, healthy and hydrating for the body. It's safe to say that we all know and accept this. In addition, we should be consuming about 4-5 servings of fruits each day.

However, combining fruits with other things such as proteins, carbohydrates and fats may not be good. It may wreak havoc with our digestive system.

So, when should we be consuming 4-5 servings of fruits? Fruits should be consumed on an empty stomach. Fruits should not be mixed with proteins, carbohydrates or fats.

It's not uncommon for us to eat fruits as desserts after a large meal. But eating fruits after a large meal may not be the best for digestion. Why? Because the fruits will not digest and ferment in your stomach.

There is a saying that "An apple a day may keep the doctor away." Just don't eat the apple after a large meal, because the doctor may return.

What is my practice of eating fruits? Since I don't have lots of time to eat fruits during my busy day, I normally would consume fruits at breakfast time.

Every morning, after drinking a glass of water upon waking, I would have my daily intake of fruits. For instance, for Mondays, Wednesdays and Fridays, I would eat a banana. For Tuesdays, Thursdays and Saturdays, I'll mix up the fruits by choosing a different one just to have a variety. I may choose other fruits on these days such as oranges, raspberries or grapes.

Not all fruits are created the same. There are different categories of fruits. Some fruits fall into the sweet category, while others are acidic.

Some fruits are in between and are labeled as sub-acidic. It is wise not to mix the different categories of fruits together.

It is best to stick with one category of fruits. For instance, when I'm at the mall, and purchase a fruit smoothie, I'll try to stick to one fruit or category of fruit and not mix them.

For instance, in the past, I would order a Banana Strawberry smoothie. Now, I will order either a Banana Smoothie or a Strawberry Smoothie. It is easier for the body to digest one type of fruit at one time.

In the past, my stomach never had a problem digesting different types of fruits consumed at one time. But over the course of the years, I've noticed that combining different categories of fruits can make the stomach work much harder.

Don't eat fruit for dessert. If you're going to eat fruit, make sure to wait a few hours.

Fruit digests the quickest. It passes through the stomach in a matter of twenty to thirty minutes. Eating fruit for dessert will cause a traffic jam in your digestive tract. The fruit will sit on top of whatever else is in your stomach and begin to ferment. By the time it reaches your intestines, there will be barely any nutrients left to absorb. This will leave you feeling bloated and tired.

Fruit is best eaten first thing in the day, or with green veggies. After twenty minutes, you can follow it up with a protein or starch.

The fourth category of fruits is the melons. When eating melons, it is best to consume melons by itself, and not with any other fruits, or foods.

Here are the different categories of fruits:

Sweet fruits
Bananas, Grapes, Dried Fruits, Dates, Raisins, Prunes, and Figs.

Acidic Fruits
Lemon, Orange, Raspberries, Pineapple, Blackberries, Kumquat, Sour Apples, Lime, Tangerines, Pomegranates, Grapefruit, Strawberries, Sour Plums.

Sub-Acidic fruits
Apples, cherries, Tart Grapes, Huckleberries, Kiwi, Papaya, Peach, Pears, Nectarines, Mangoes, Sweet Plums, Apricots, Fresh figs.

Melons
Cantaloupe, Honey Dew, Watermelon, Casaba, Musk, Persian, Crenshaw

Step IV

Do not combine Protein with Starch

This is one of the most important steps in food combinations. Do not combine protein with starch.

Yes, I know. Protein and starch, together, is a staple of the American diet. It is the standard for most of us.

Most of us love our hamburgers, hot-dogs and pizzas. But this typical American diet is combining protein with starch.

The standard Asian diet is the same. They combine a bowl of rice with their favorite beef, chicken or pork dish. My favorite Japanese dish is Teriyaki Chicken. My favorite Vietnamese dish is Pho. I thought that these foods were overall healthy, but then I realize that it is combining protein with starch. Again, my stomach used to digest these food combinations just fine, and I had no problem staying thin and healthy.

I realized that protein and starch digest differently. Both types of food need a different stomach environment to digest.

Proteins need an acidic environment in the stomach. Starches digest much better in an alkaline environment. The contrasting environments within the digestive system neutralize each other. This will likely leave you feeling bloated and full of gas.

Below are the types of starches and proteins. Remember, although it is a standard American diet to combine protein and starch, but they don't digest very well together.

Starches
pasta, potatoes, corn, breads, popcorn, crackers, tortillas, cereals, rice, oatmeal, barley, millet and other grains.

Protein
Meat, fish, milk, soybeans, nuts, olives, fowl, eggs, cheese, yogurt, seeds, coconut.

Step V

Don't combine protein with another type of protein

Just as it is important not to combine protein with starch, it is also important not to combine different types of protein together.

Why? Because different types of proteins takes a different amounts of time for digestion.

For instance, an egg may take a hour to digest. Fish may take about 3-4 hours to digest. Red Meat or Pork, or seafood may take even longer to digest.

It's better to stick with one type of protein per meal. I don't know about you, but I love surf and turf.

For the sake of good health and weight loss, I also had to bid farewell to surf and turf.

Step VI

Don't Drink Water During the Meal

Many of us when dining, normally would have a sip of water between each bite. This is not uncommon.

But drinking water during the meal may slow down digestion and dilute digestive enzymes in the stomach. It's not that drinking water is bad for you.

I recommend that you try drinking a glass of water half-hour before each meal to help stimulate stomach digestion.

Wait for about an hour after each meal to drink another glass of water.

Step VII

Thus far, most of the food suggestions have been focused on digestion within the stomach.

Digestion, however, doesn't just begin in the stomach. Digestion begins in the mouth.

If the food has been properly broken down in the mouth, it will be less work for the stomach.

That's why it is utmost important to chew your foods well. Try to chew your food thoroughly before you swallow.

Growing up in a poor family with four brothers, I remembered that I had to devour my food quickly, otherwise I would starve.

That bad habit has been with me over the years. I could eat a fast food value meal in just a few minutes. Eating used to be a contest for me.

Dining at meals should not be a contest. The food must be enjoyed and savored.

One time, I was overseas, and visited Paris. I noticed that families over there would spend a few hours at meals.

Here in America, we don't have the luxury of time because of our busy schedules. But it's not an excuse to swallow food without properly chewing the food.

Take time with your food, and savor the taste by chewing your food thoroughly. Your stomach will thank you for it!

Step VIII

If we can't combine different types of fruits, or combine proteins, fats and vegetables, what certain kinds of food combinations are acceptable?

Acceptable food combinations is any type of foods with vegetables. Vegetables are considered neutral types of food and can be mixed with fats, carbohydrates or proteins.

It is recommended to have vegetables at every meal. It will help your digestive system. Below are the types of vegetables that can be combined with all types of foods.

VEGETABLES:

◊ Asparagus,
◊ Beet greens,
◊ Broccoli,
◊ Brussels Sprouts,
◊ Cabbage,
◊ Celery,
◊ Chard,
◊ Chicory,
◊ Collards,
◊ Cucumber,
◊ Dandelion,

- ◊ Eggplant,
- ◊ Endive,
- ◊ Escarole,
- ◊ Garlic,
- ◊ Green Beans,
- ◊ Kale,
- ◊ Kohlrabi,
- ◊ Leeks,
- ◊ Lettuce,
- ◊ Mushrooms,
- ◊ Onions,
- ◊ Parsley,
- ◊ Radishes,
- ◊ Scallions,
- ◊ Spinach,
- ◊ Sprouts,
- ◊ Squash,
- ◊ Sweet Pepper,
- ◊ Tomatoes,
- ◊ Turnips,
- ◊ Watercress,
- ◊ Zucchini

Step IX

Now, I need to address the fats category.

In our current society, Fats are considered an evil and to be avoided. So many foods today are advertised as Fat-Free or Low-Fat.

But not all types of fats are the same. These advertisements are more about trans-fat which to be avoided completely.

Healthy fats (not trans-fat) are good for the body, especially for hair, skin, and nails. With that being said, it's also good to limit your fats because they could slow down your digestion.

For instance, use small amounts of olive oil. When consuming avocados, a few slices will suffice.

When combining proteins with fats, the fats inhibits the enzymes needed for protein digestion, so it's best keep the distance between the two.

However, fats (like avocados and oils) and carbohydrates mix well, and the former also play nicely with leafy greens.

Treat foods that are considered both proteins and fat (cheese, seeds, nuts) as proteins.

Don't eat Avocado with Nuts. An avocado is a fat, combined with nuts which is a protein. The fat properties of the avocado have an inhibiting effect of the digestion of the protein in nuts.

Do not combine olive oil with nuts. Olive oil and nuts are commonly combined in pesto and salad dressings. Olive oil is a fat and nuts are proteins. Again, the fat has an inhibiting effect of the digestion of the protein.

Below are the list of types of fats.

◊ Butter,
◊ cream,
◊ corn oil,
◊ olive oil,
◊ safflower oil,
◊ sunflower oil,
◊ avocado,
◊ lard,
◊ nut oils,
◊ soy oil,
◊ sesame oil.

Step X

All of these guidelines may seem overwhelming to you at first. It did for me because I wasn't familiar with it.

I shared these food combination ideas with my parents, siblings and close friends. Some of them were believers and some were not. Some thought I was just being crazy. But the results speak for itself, and many people over time became believers because of my own weight loss.

These combination rules may be seem very difficult at first. But over time, like everything else, practice makes perfect. Proper food combinations will become second-nature.

Sometimes, on certain days, maybe once a week, it's acceptable to have a cheat meal where the guidelines doesn't have to be followed. That could change things up for the body, and it is good and healthy for the body to do something different.

Given that there are many guidelines to follow, the general idea is that we should keep it simple for our stomachs.

You can use the 80/20 rule which is to consume 80% vegetable with a 20% side of anything else such as protein, carbohydrates, or fats. As long as we choose one of the food categories, and do not combine proteins, carbohydrates or fats.

Here is a chart that you could refer to, just in case you forget.

Food Combining Chart for Good Digestion

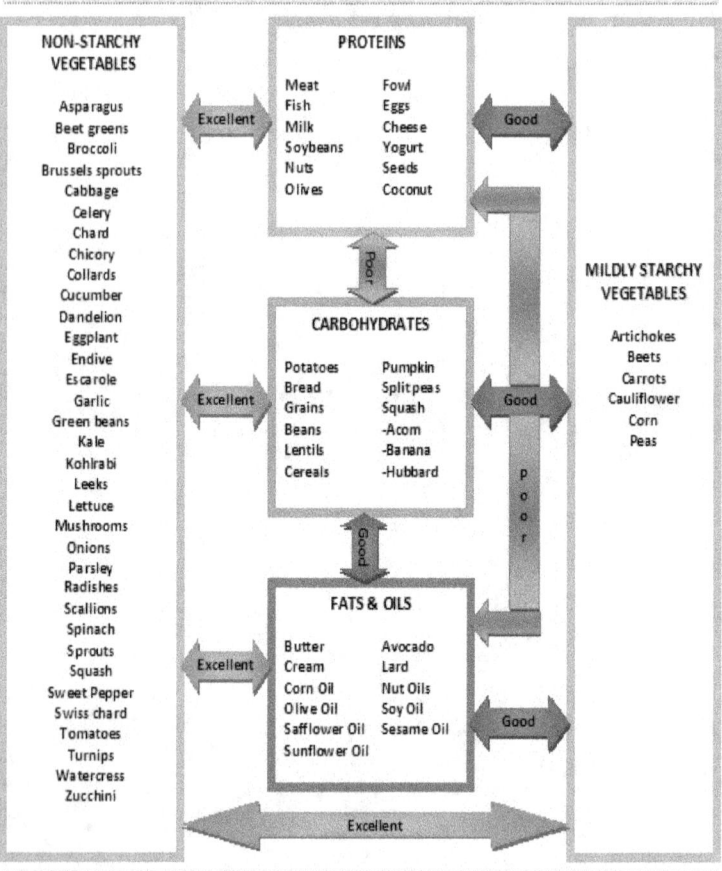

NON-STARCHY VEGETABLES

Asparagus
Beet greens
Broccoli
Brussels sprouts
Cabbage
Celery
Chard
Chicory
Collards
Cucumber
Dandelion
Eggplant
Endive
Escarole
Garlic
Green beans
Kale
Kohlrabi
Leeks
Lettuce
Mushrooms
Onions
Parsley
Radishes
Scallions
Spinach
Sprouts
Squash
Sweet Pepper
Swiss chard
Tomatoes
Turnips
Watercress
Zucchini

PROTEINS

Meat	Fowl
Fish	Eggs
Milk	Cheese
Soybeans	Yogurt
Nuts	Seeds
Olives	Coconut

CARBOHYDRATES

Potatoes	Pumpkin
Bread	Split peas
Grains	Squash
Beans	-Acorn
Lentils	-Banana
Cereals	-Hubbard

FATS & OILS

Butter	Avocado
Cream	Lard
Corn Oil	Nut Oils
Olive Oil	Soy Oil
Safflower Oil	Sesame Oil
Sunflower Oil	

MILDLY STARCHY VEGETABLES

Artichokes
Beets
Carrots
Cauliflower
Corn
Peas

Excellent — Good — Poor — Good — poor — Excellent

Fruits are best when eaten separate from other foods on an empty stomach. It is best to eat melons and sweet fruits separately. Fruit makes an awesome breakfast and an energetic start to the day.

ACID FRUITS		SUB ACID FRUITS		SWEET FRUITS		MELONS
Lemon	Lime	Apples	Pears	Bananas	Raisins	Cantaloupe
Orange	Tangerines	Cherries	Nectarines	Grapes	Prunes	Honey dew
Raspberries	Pomegranate	Tart Grapes	Mangoes	Dried fruits	Figs	Watermelon
Pineapple	Grapefruit	Huckleberries	Sweet Plums	Dates		Casaba
Blackberries	Strawberries	Kiwi	Apricots			Musk
Kumquat	Sour Plums	Papaya	Fresh Figs			Persian
Sour apples		Peach				Crenshaw